Heather's Story For God's Glory

This little book will give you a peek into the life of
Heather Cape throughout the last 30 years.
As a healthy 9 year old little girl,
her life would change greatly
on July 15, 1994!

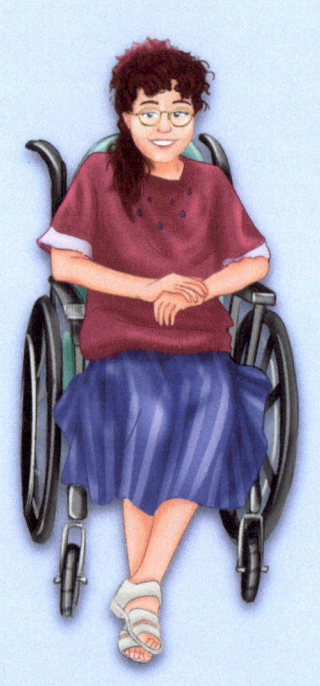 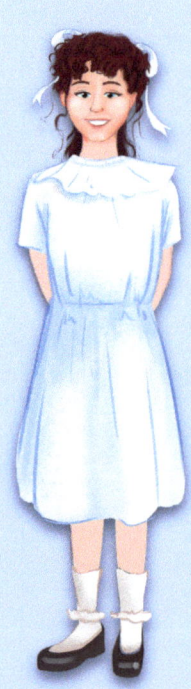 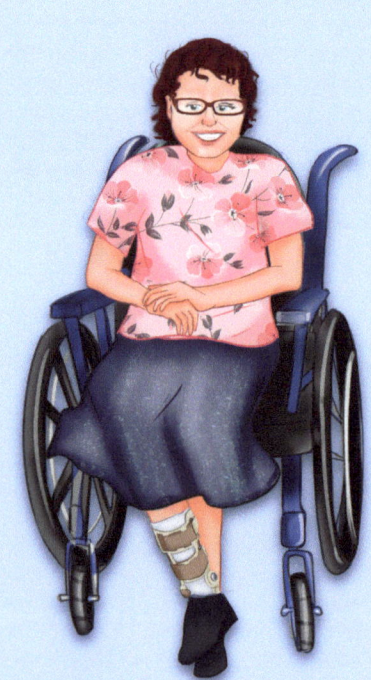

Dedication

Heather Cape has needed medical care since she was 9 years old. God has been very good to always take care of her.

This book is dedicated to the hundreds of medical professionals who have assisted us in giving her care. Also included in this dedication are her two sisters, Jenah and Hannah who are illustrated in this book as well, and who have always supported and loved their sister unconditionally.

Each one of you have had a huge part in helping restore her health to a "better quality of life." We are very grateful for all you have done! May God bless each of you!

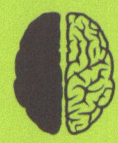

THIS I KNOW WITH HALF-OF MY BRAIN
Copyright © 2024 by Steve and Wanda Cape

All rights reserved. No part of this book may be used or reproduced or transmitted in any form whatsoever without written permission from the author.

For more information, please contact:
Cerebrum Connections
5750 Antonio Lane
Hixson, TN 37343
Cerebrumconnections@gmail.com
Godmakesnomistakes.com

All Scripture quotations are taken from the King James Bible.

ISBN-13: 979-8-218-44538-6 (paperback)
ISBN-13: 979-8-9911558-0-9 (hardback)
ISBN-13: 979-8-9911558-1-6 (e-book)

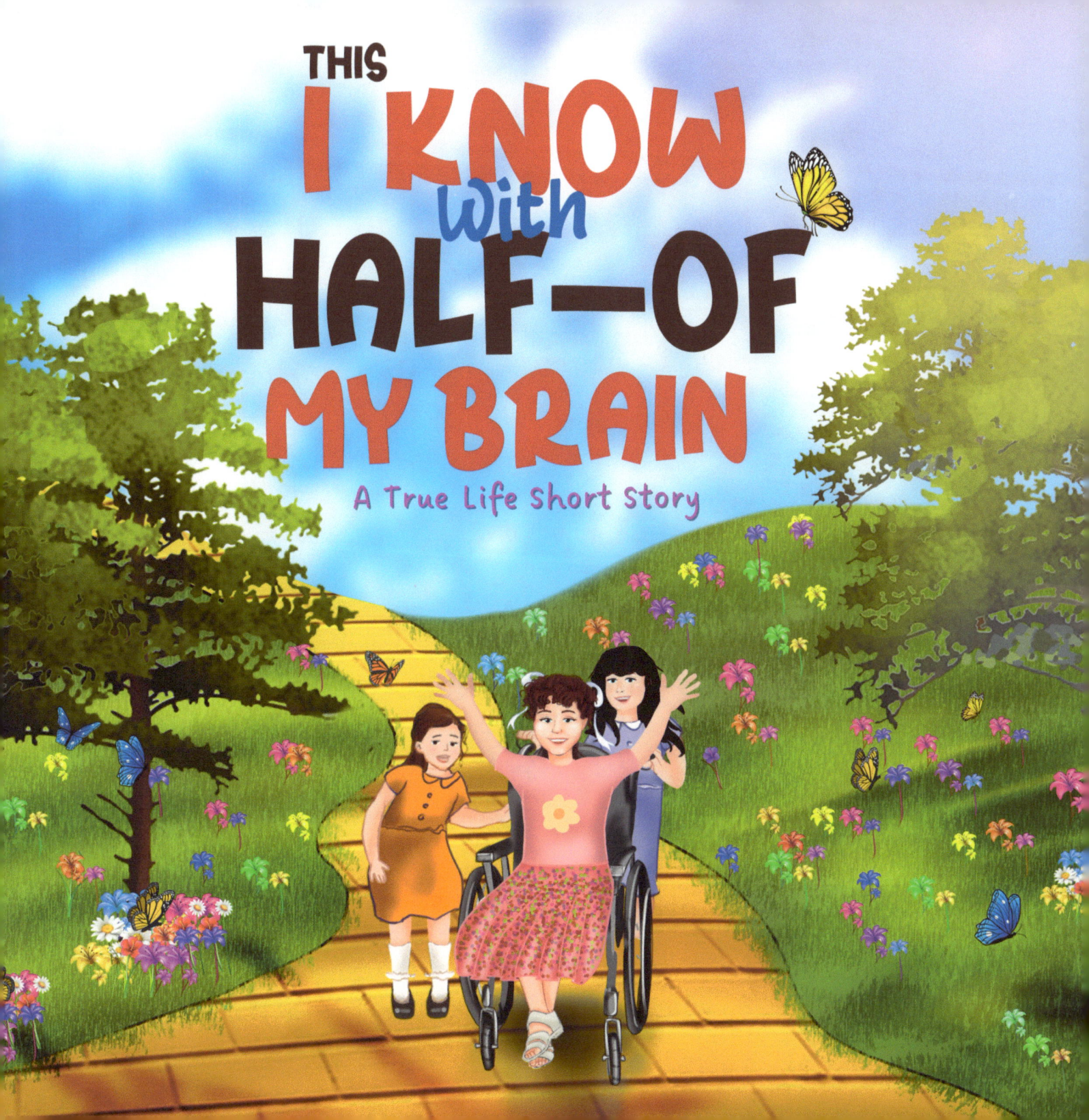

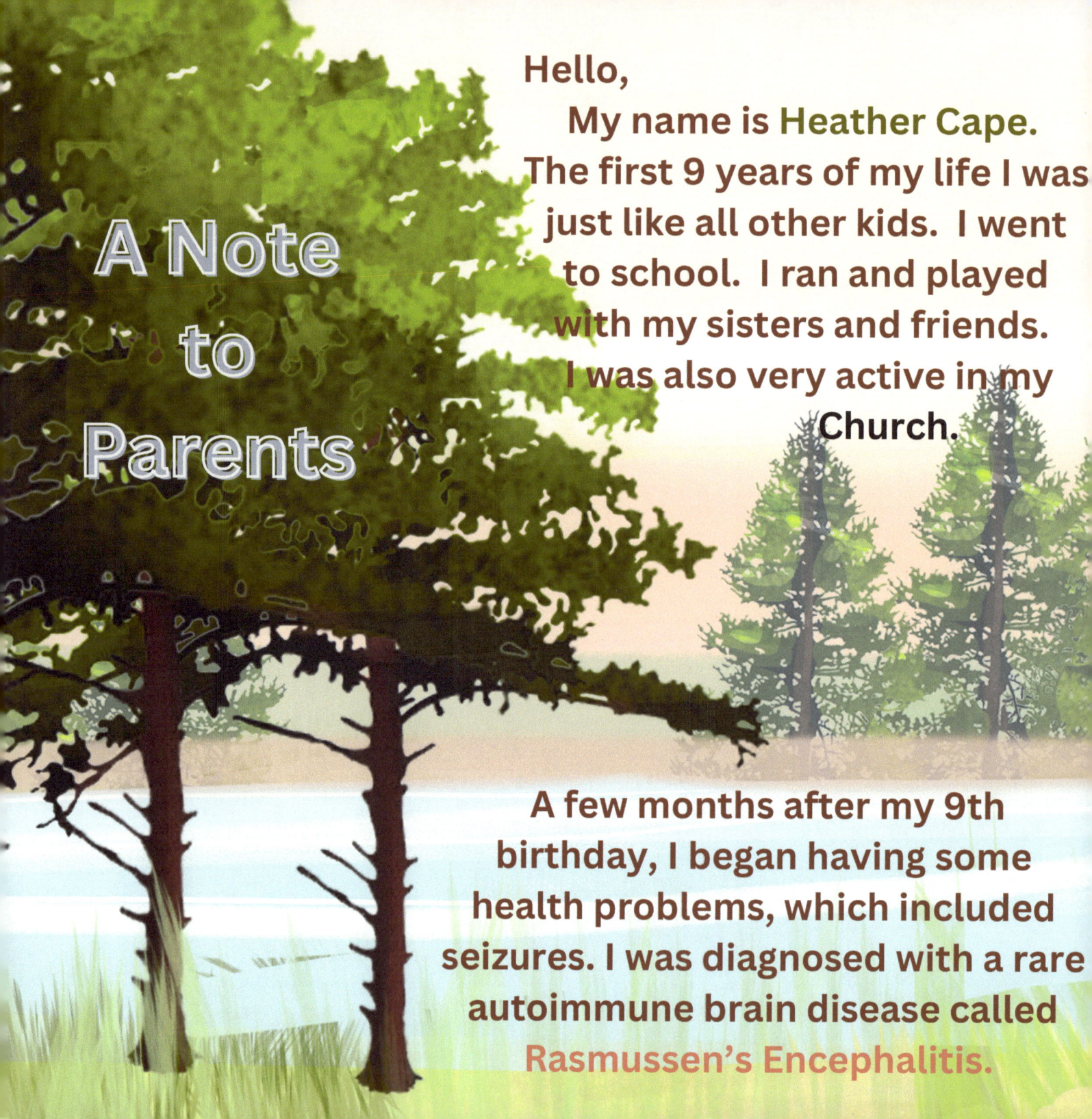

A Note to Parents

Hello,
My name is Heather Cape. The first 9 years of my life I was just like all other kids. I went to school. I ran and played with my sisters and friends. I was also very active in my Church.

A few months after my 9th birthday, I began having some health problems, which included seizures. I was diagnosed with a rare autoimmune brain disease called Rasmussen's Encephalitis.

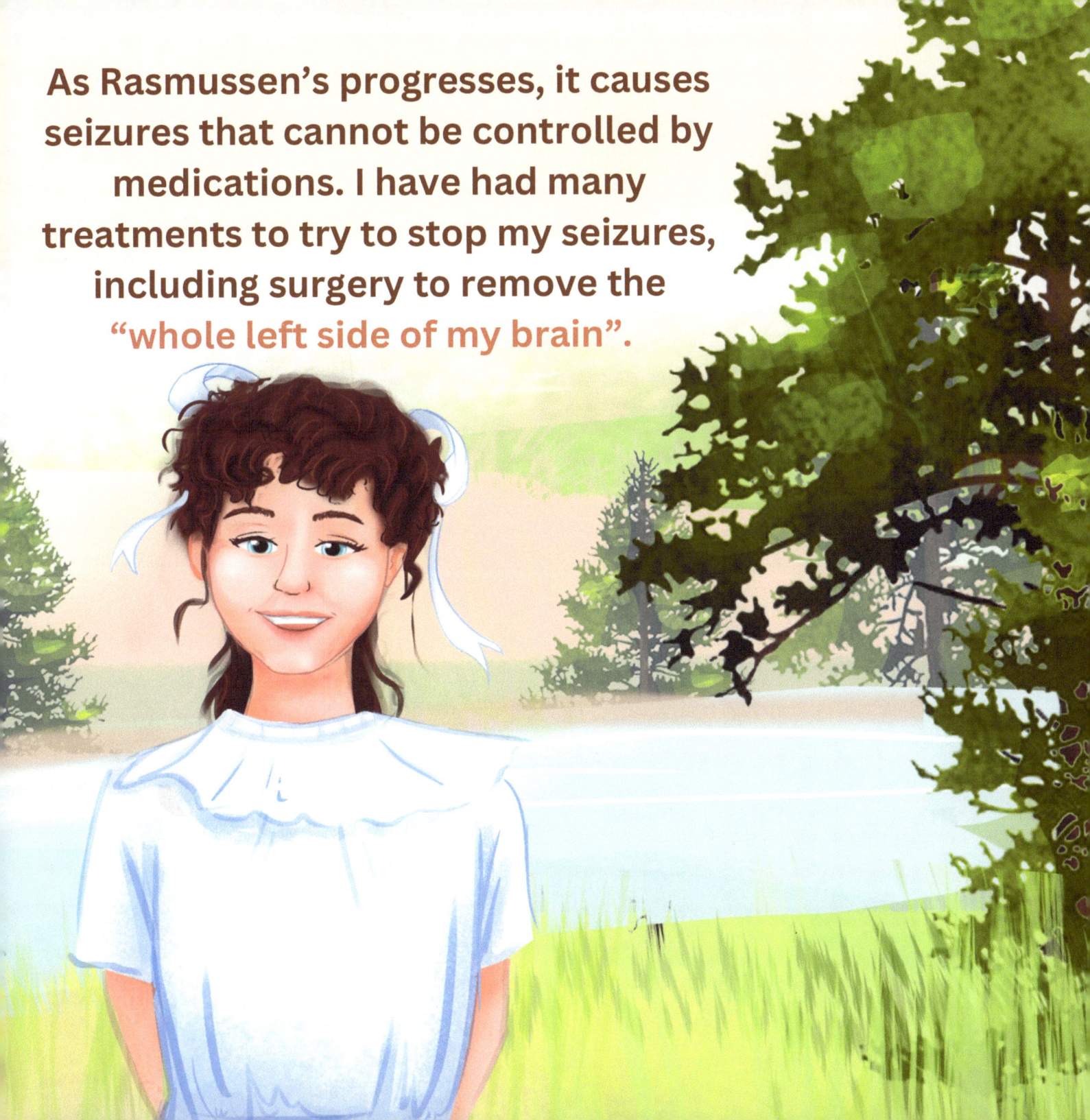

As Rasmussen's progresses, it causes seizures that cannot be controlled by medications. I have had many treatments to try to stop my seizures, including surgery to remove the "whole left side of my brain".

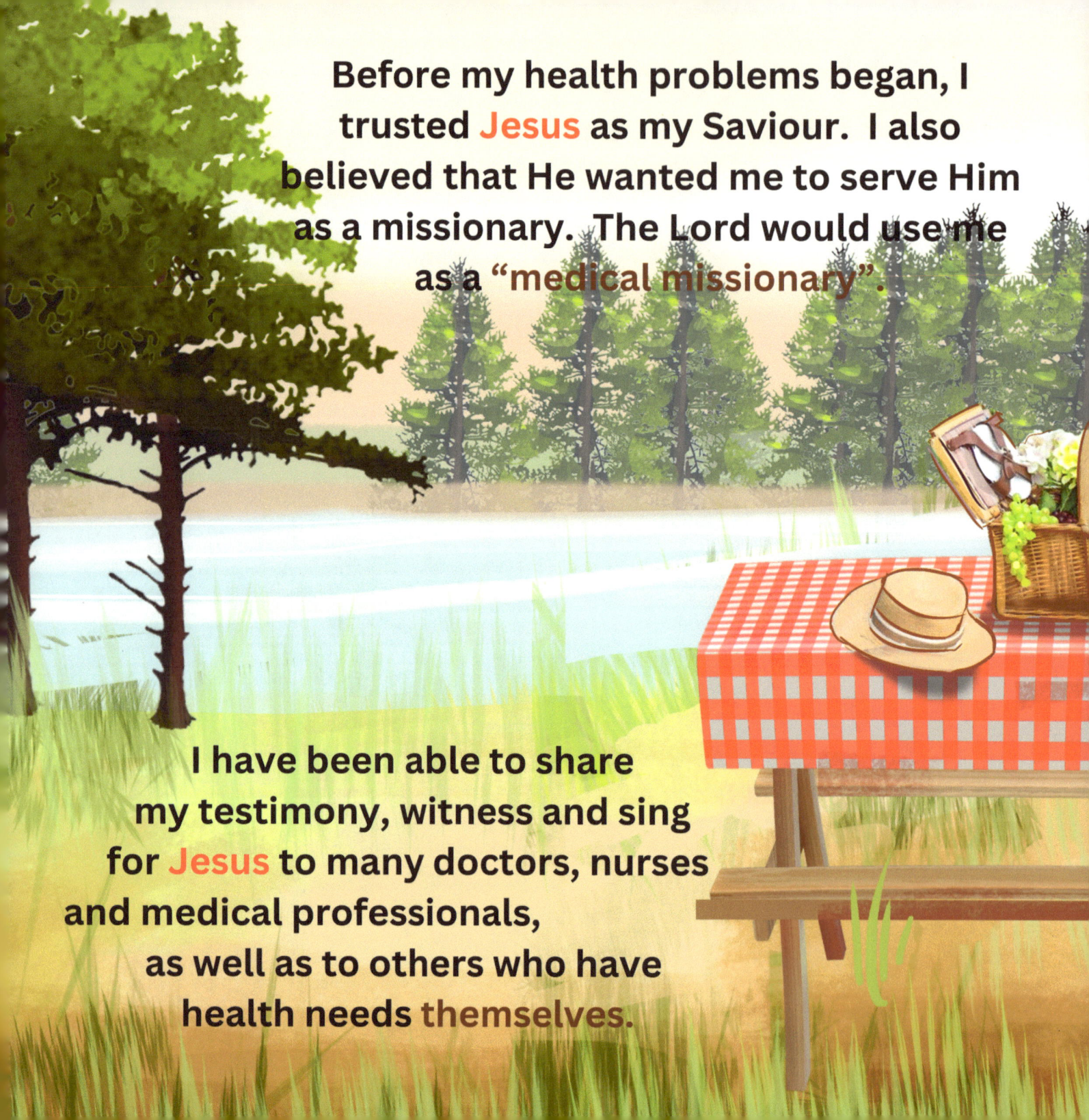

Before my health problems began, I trusted Jesus as my Saviour. I also believed that He wanted me to serve Him as a missionary. The Lord would use me as a "medical missionary".

I have been able to share my testimony, witness and sing for Jesus to many doctors, nurses and medical professionals, as well as to others who have health needs themselves.

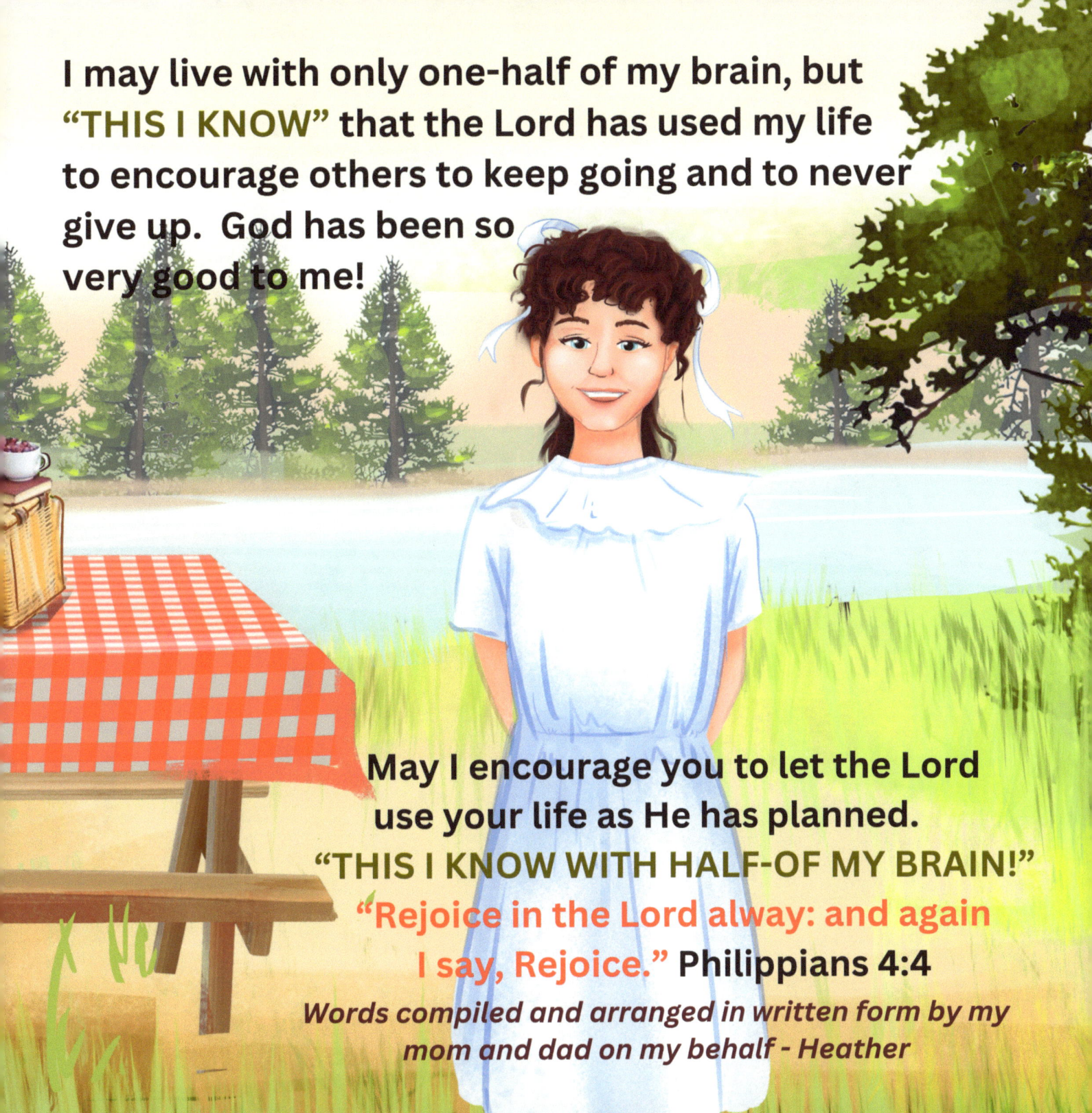

I may live with only one-half of my brain, but "THIS I KNOW" that the Lord has used my life to encourage others to keep going and to never give up. God has been so very good to me!

May I encourage you to let the Lord use your life as He has planned. "THIS I KNOW WITH HALF-OF MY BRAIN!" "Rejoice in the Lord alway: and again I say, Rejoice." Philippians 4:4

Words compiled and arranged in written form by my mom and dad on my behalf - Heather

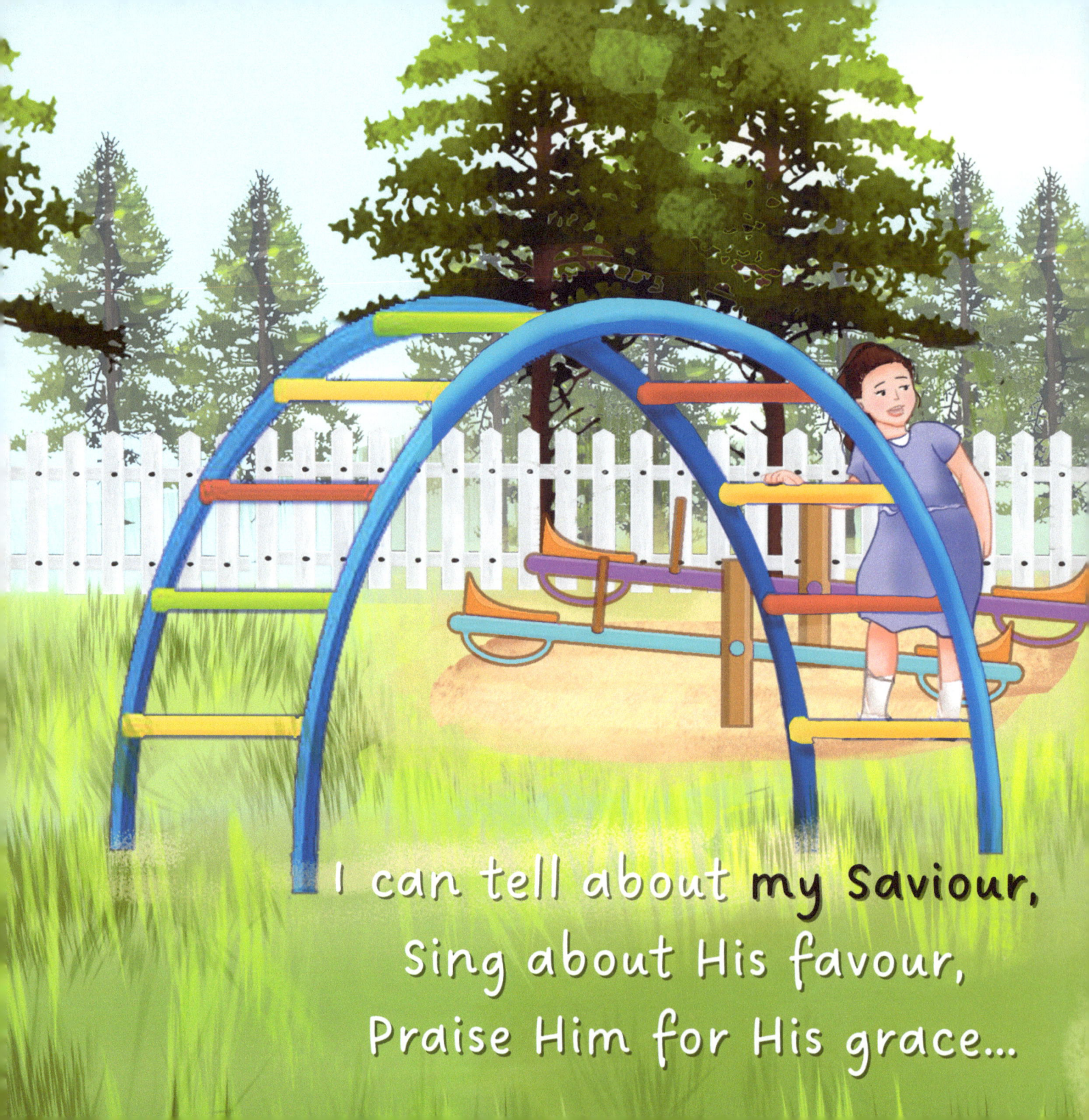

I can tell about my Saviour,
Sing about His favour,
Praise Him for His grace...

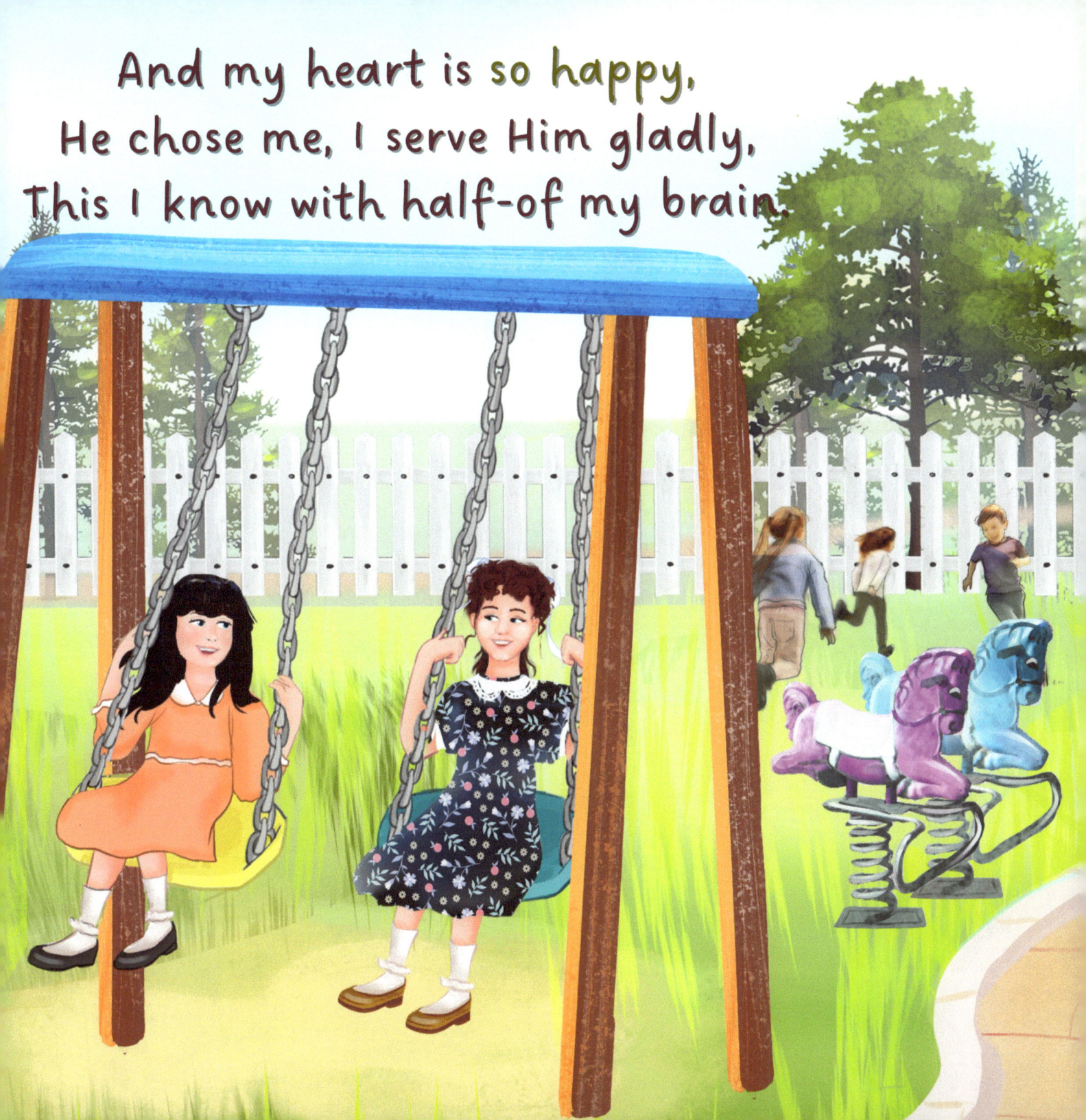
And my heart is so happy,
He chose me, I serve Him gladly,
This I know with half-of my brain.

I could wish away my illness,
Cry and never witness,
Be miserably depressed...

"But this would be oh, so worthless,
For my life which has a purpose,
To bring glory to His Name.

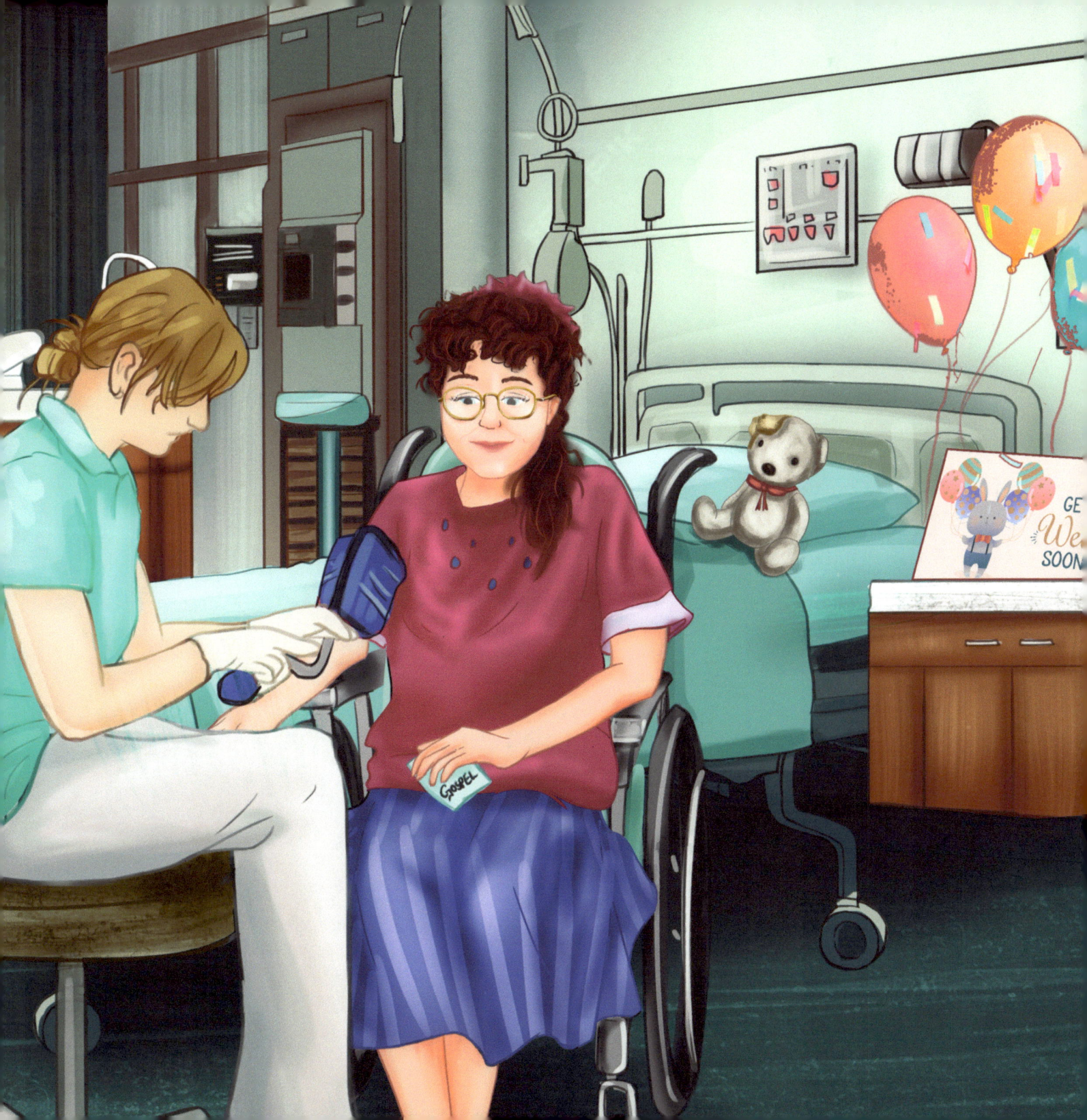

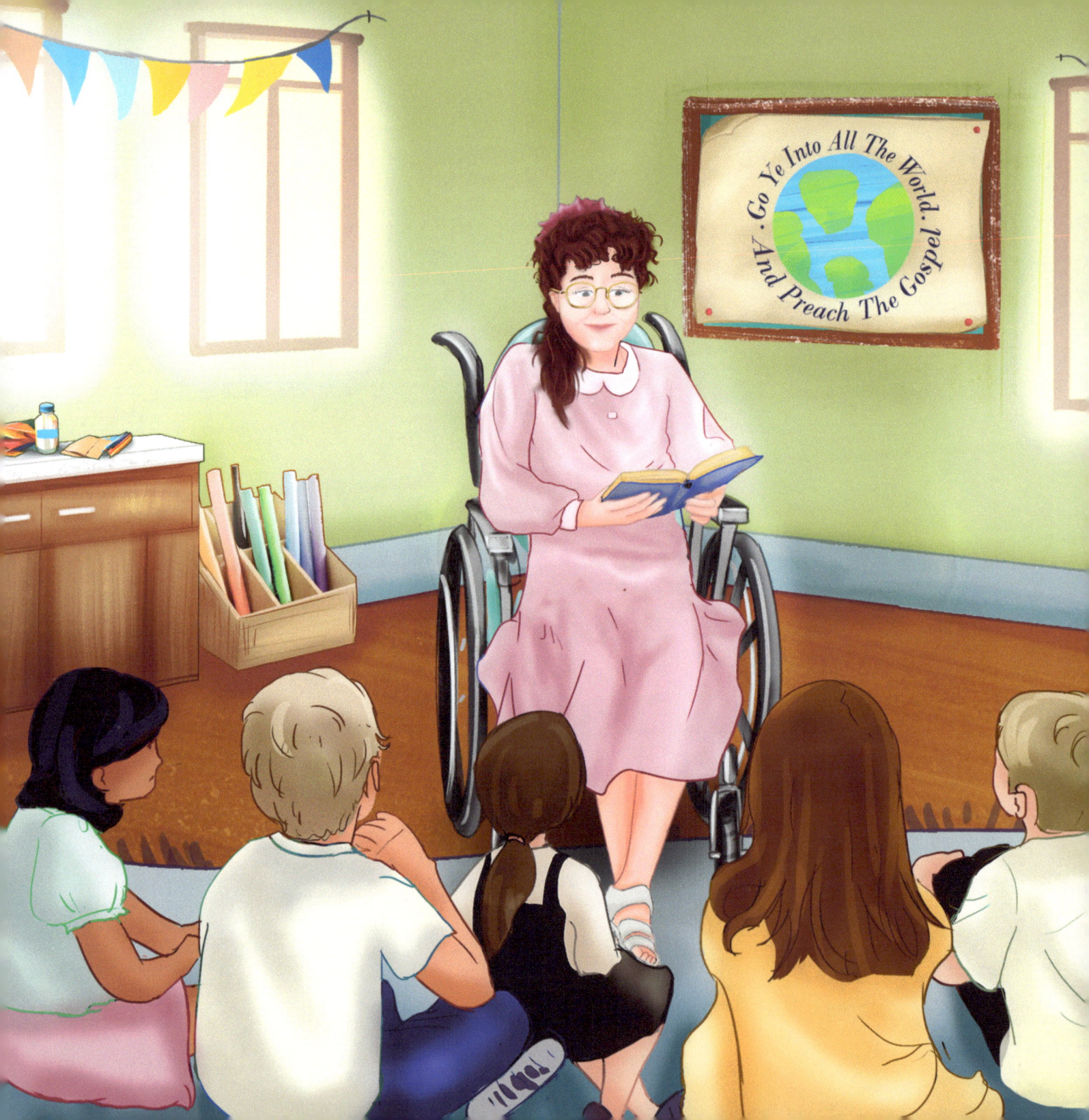

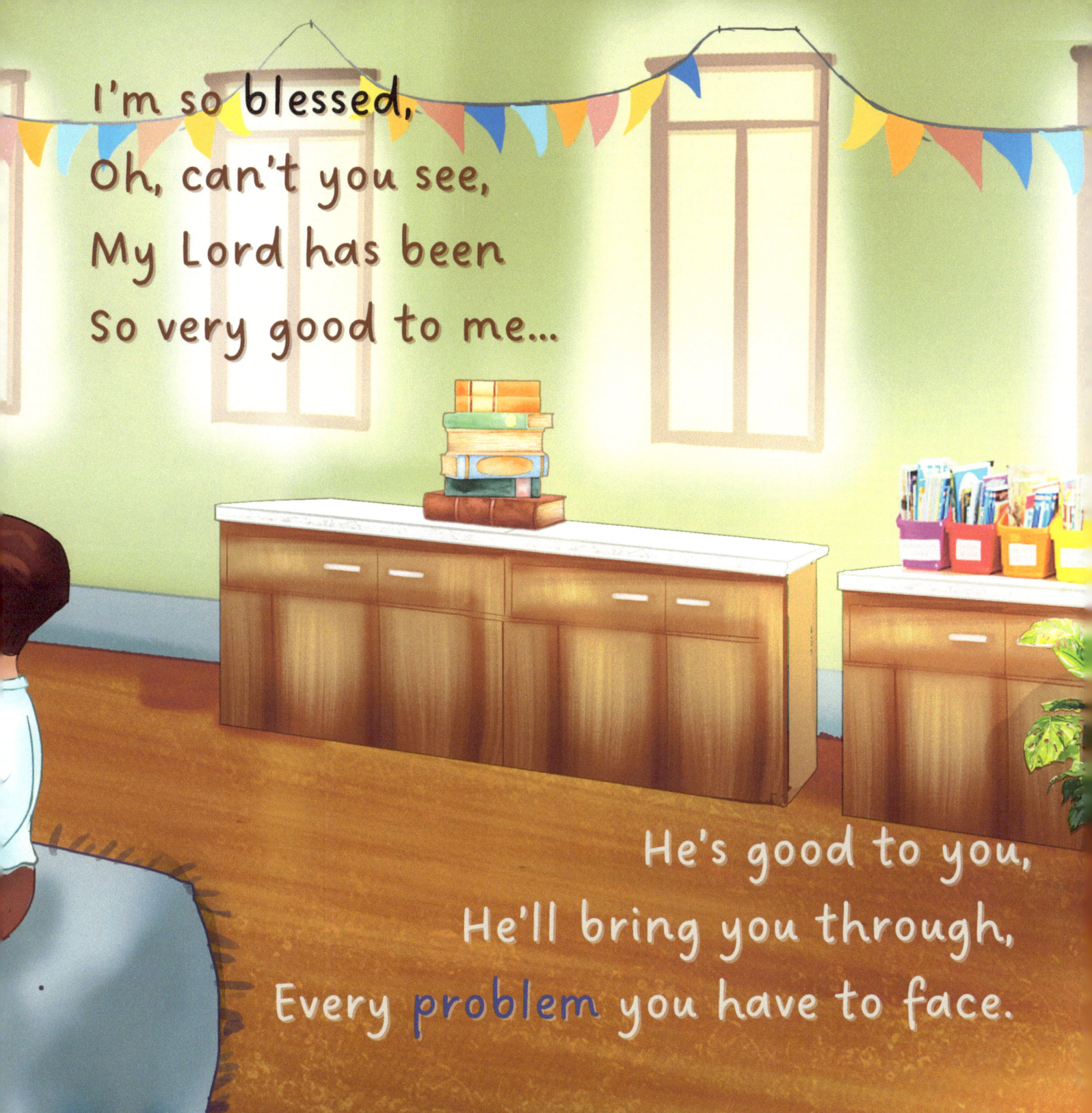

I'm so blessed,
Oh, can't you see,
My Lord has been
So very good to me...

He's good to you,
He'll bring you through,
Every problem you have to face.

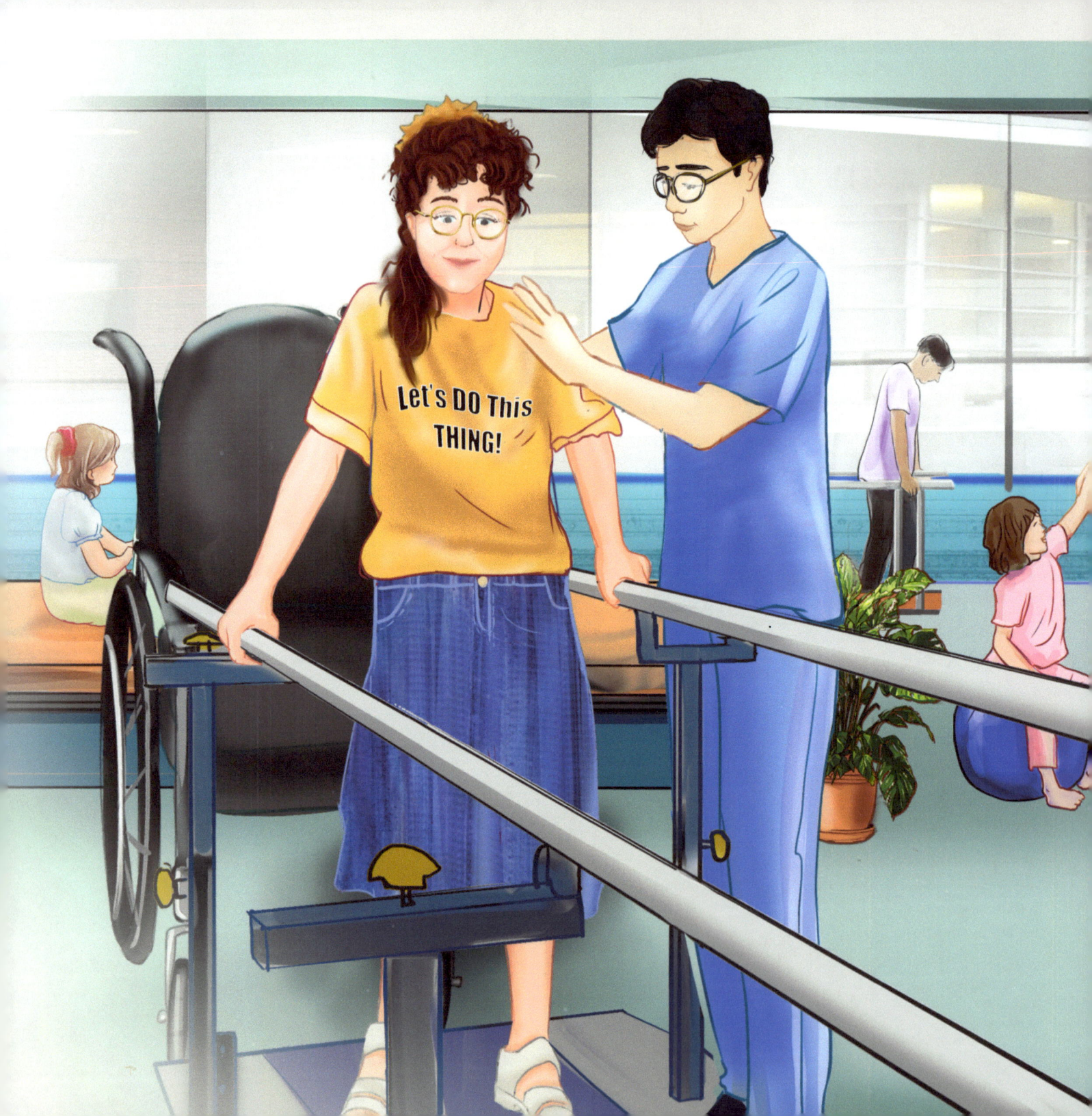

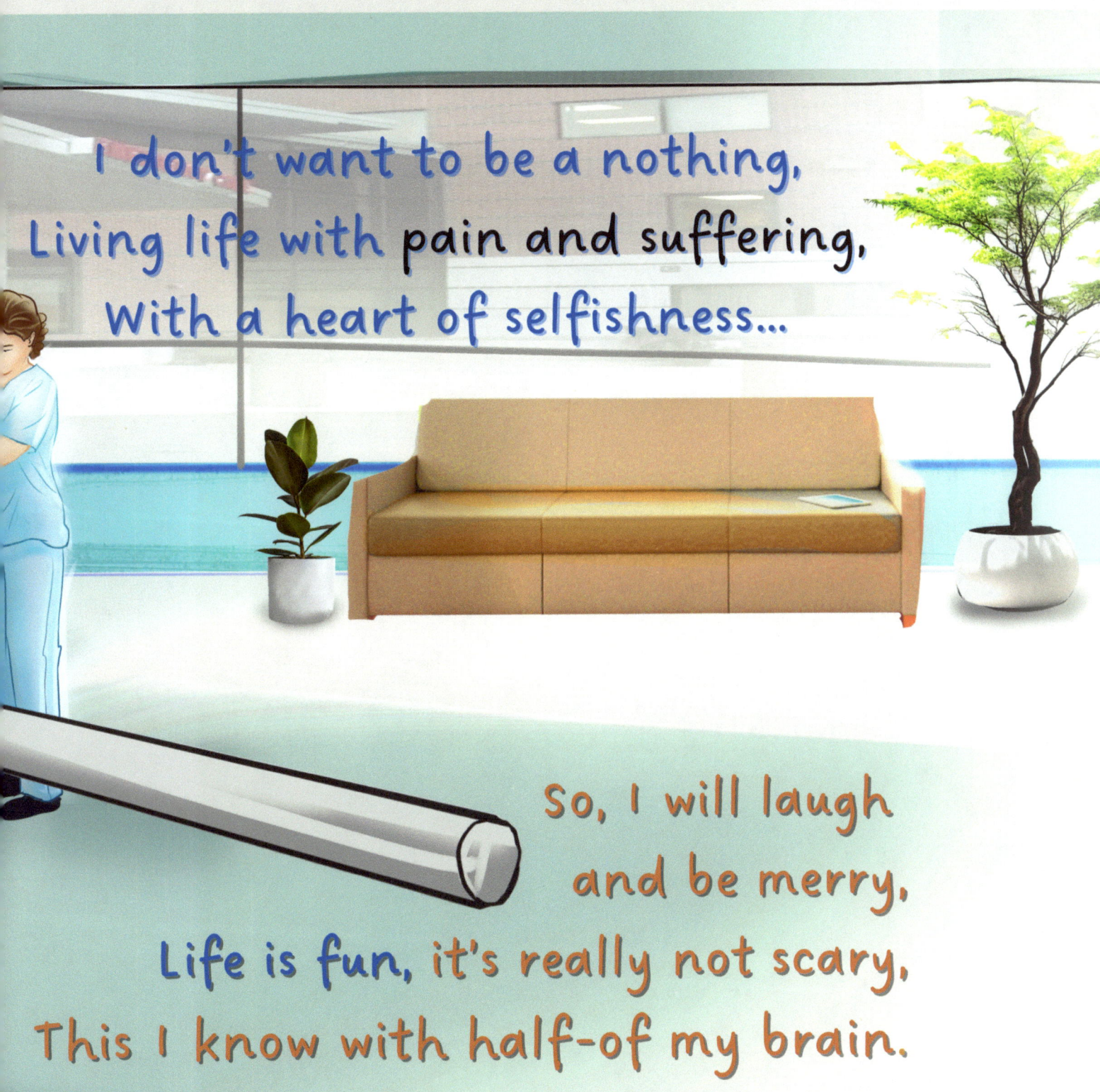

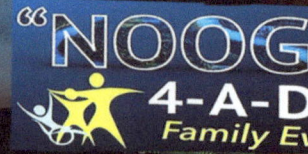

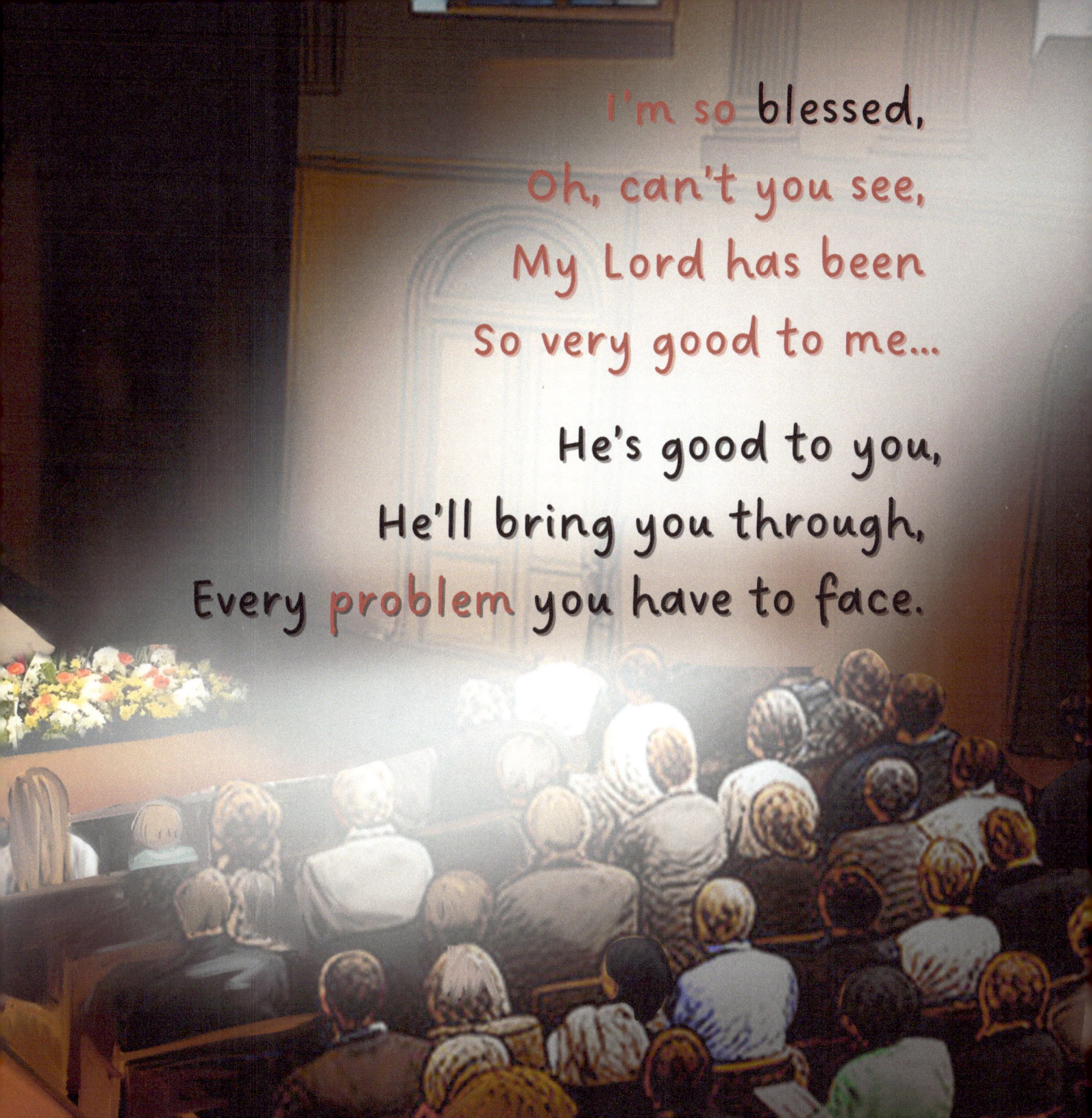

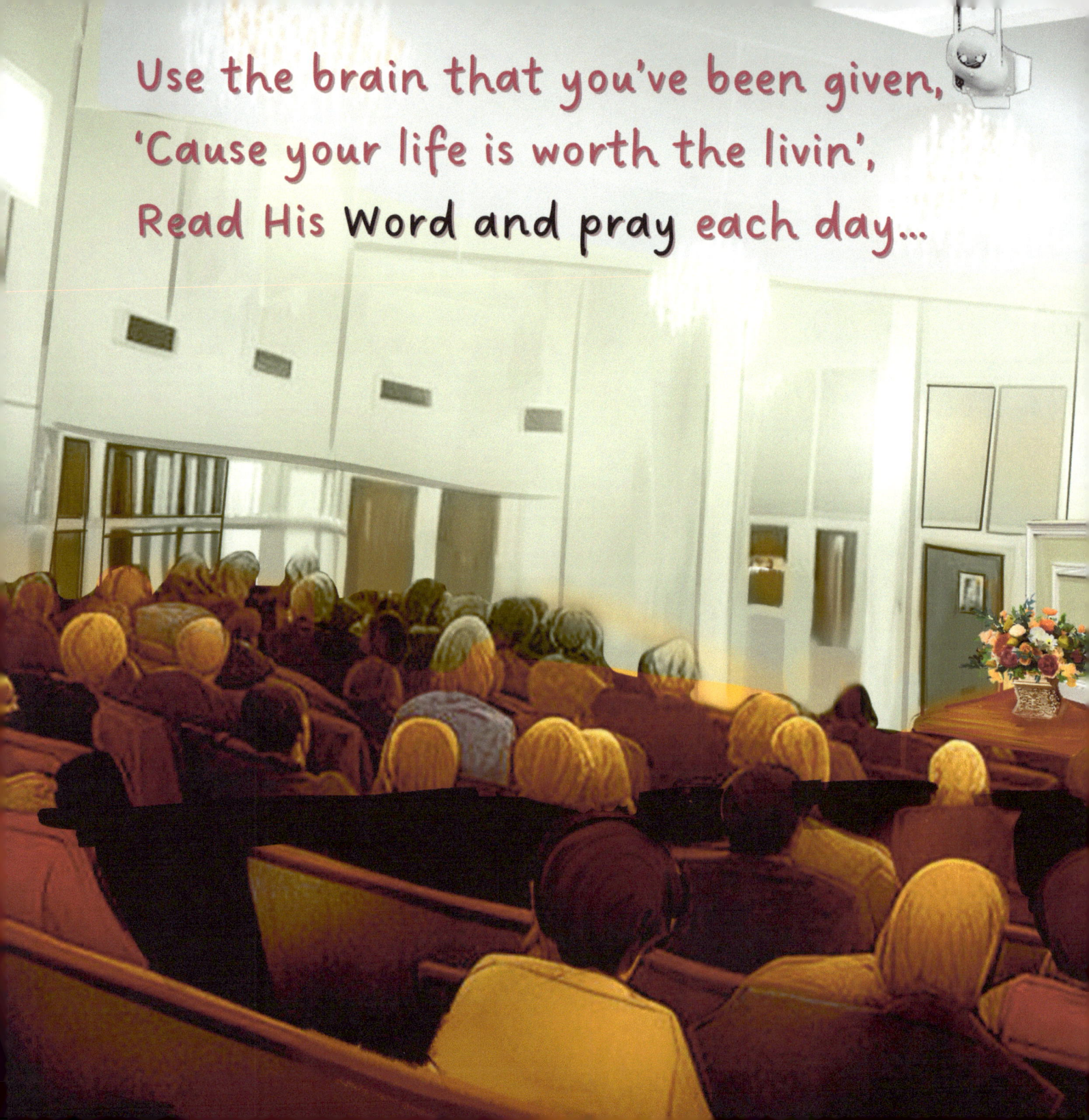

Use the brain that you've been given,
'Cause your life is worth the livin',
Read His Word and pray each day...

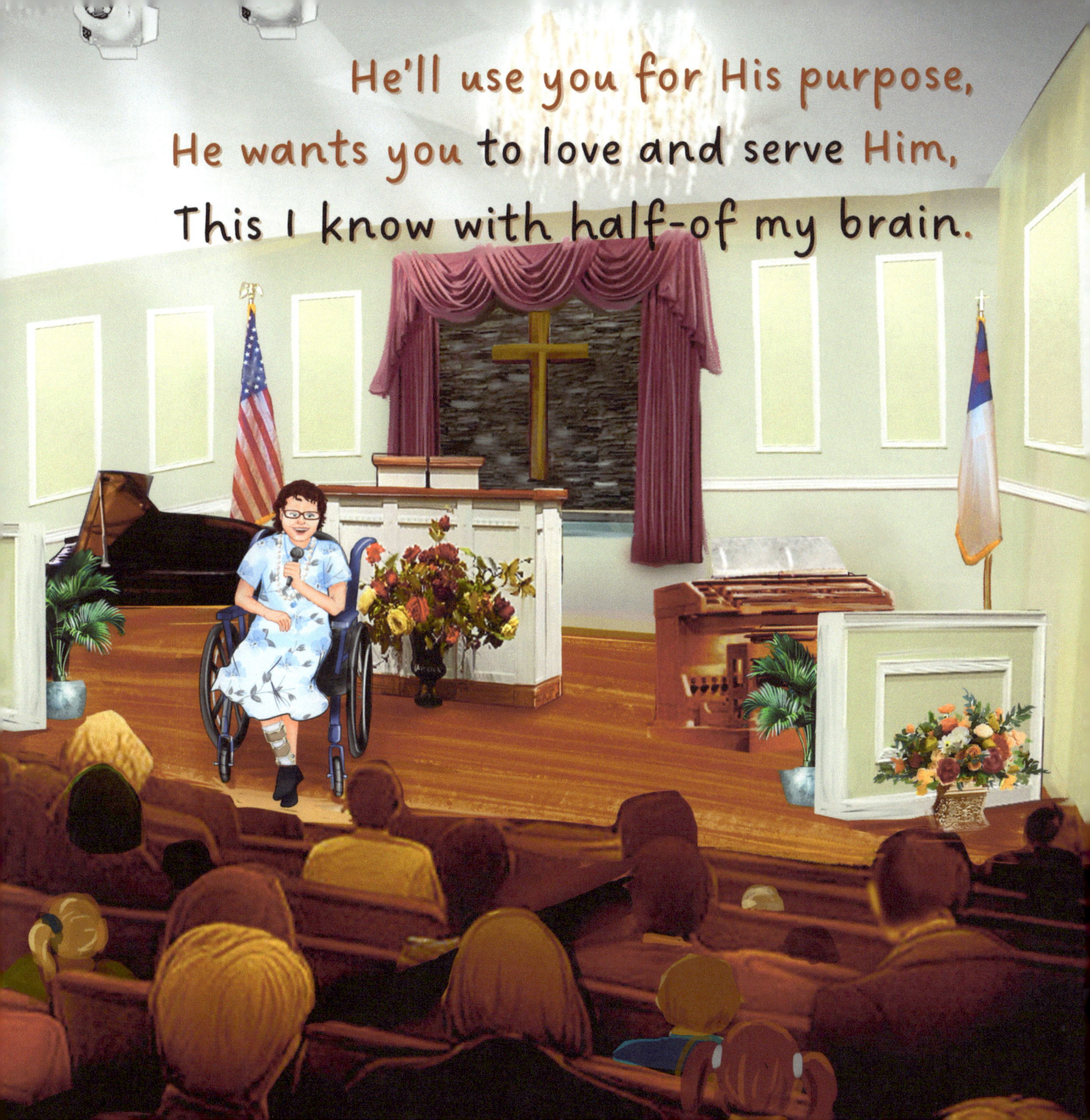

A Note from the Authors

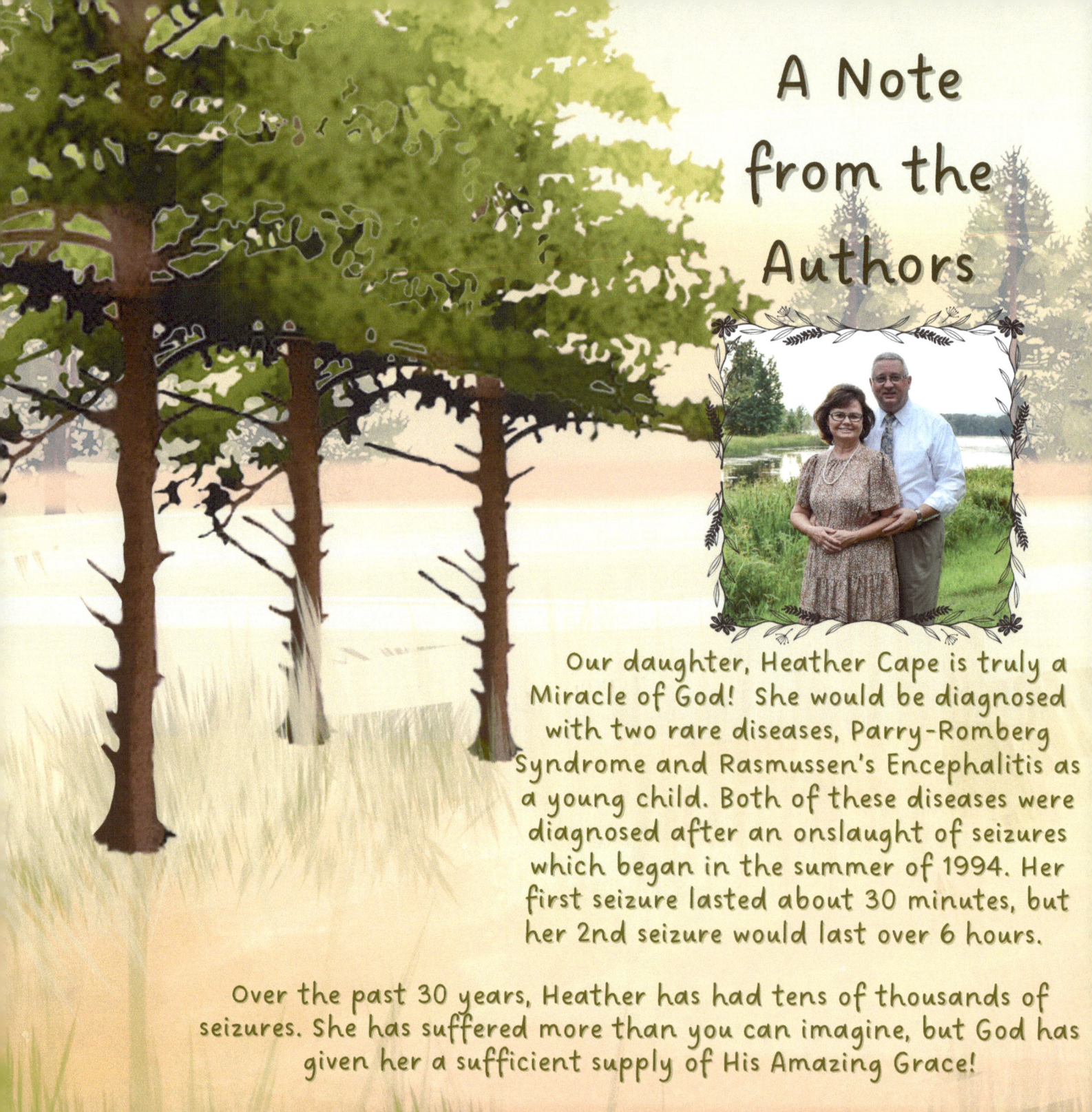

Our daughter, Heather Cape is truly a Miracle of God! She would be diagnosed with two rare diseases, Parry-Romberg Syndrome and Rasmussen's Encephalitis as a young child. Both of these diseases were diagnosed after an onslaught of seizures which began in the summer of 1994. Her first seizure lasted about 30 minutes, but her 2nd seizure would last over 6 hours.

Over the past 30 years, Heather has had tens of thousands of seizures. She has suffered more than you can imagine, but God has given her a sufficient supply of His Amazing Grace!

She views her illness as an "Opportunity" to help everyone she meets along the way. Our prayer is that this book will be an encouragement to all who read it from the youngest to the oldest. The Lord can use your challenges, no matter what they may be to help others and to bring Glory to Him.

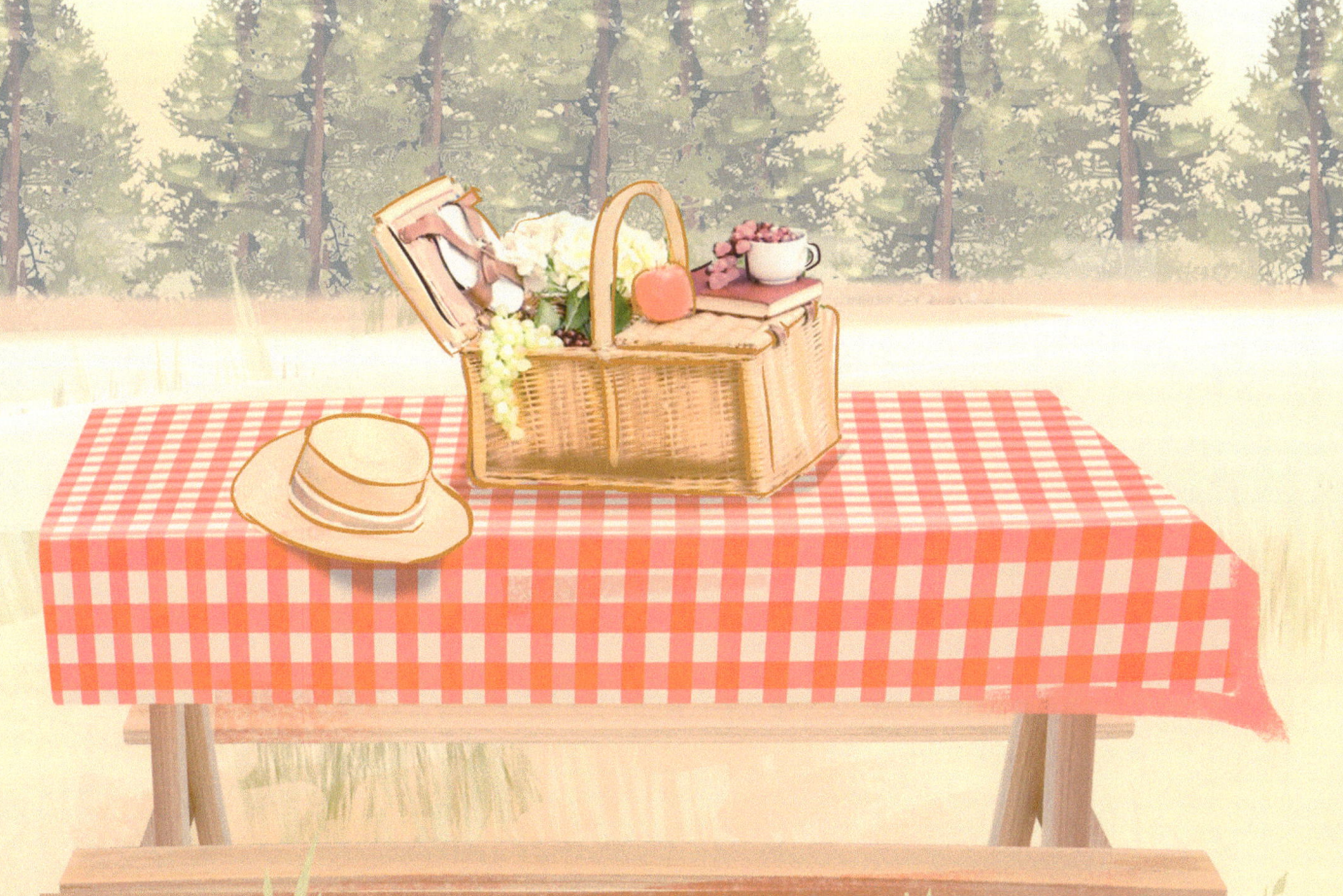

II Corinthians 12:9, "And he said unto me, My grace is sufficient for thee: for my strength is made perfect in weakness. Most gladly therefore will I rather glory in my infirmities, that the power of Christ may rest upon me."

HELPFUL TERMS

<u>Seizures</u> - A seizure is defined as a sudden, electrical discharge in the brain. A person can lose awareness and consciousness.

<u>Rasmussen's Encephalitis</u>- A rare autoimmune brain disease that affects 1 out of every 10 million people, and usually occurs in children under the age of 10. Most individuals with Rasmussen's encephalitis will experience frequent seizures and progressive brain damage in the affected hemisphere of the brain.

<u>Parry Romberg Syndrome</u>- A rare disorder that affects 1 out of every 250,000, which is characterized by slowly progressive deterioration (atrophy) of the skin and soft tissues of half of the face (hemifacial atrophy). It is more common in females than in males.

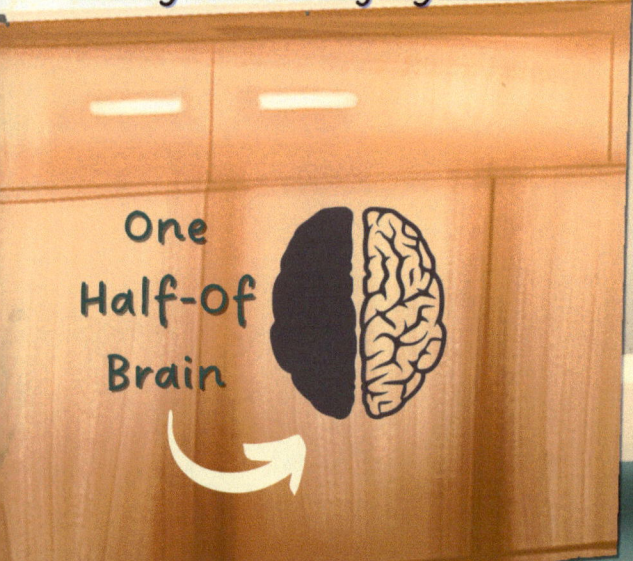

One Half-Of Brain

WHAT IS A BRAIN HEMISPHERECTOMY?

A Hemispherectomy is a rare surgery that either removes or disconnects half of the brain from the other half.

AMAZING FACTS ABOUT OUR BRAINS

- The human brain is made of mainly three parts: Cerebrum, Cerebellum, and Brain Stem.
- Cerebrum – It is the largest part of the brain. It has many wrinkles, making it look something like a walnut without its shell. It's divided into two halves, the left and right hemisphere, by a deep groove. The two hemispheres connect using a structure called the corpus callosum.
- The two hemispheres of your brain also have four main lobes each:
    - <u>Frontal</u> (at the front of your head).
    - <u>Parietal</u> (at the top of your head).
    - <u>Temporal</u> (at the side of your head).
    - <u>Occipital</u> (at the back of your head).
- It's faster than the fastest <u>computer</u>.
- It weighs about 3 pounds and uses 20% of your oxygen.
- It can't feel pain.
- It contains about 100 billion microscopic cells called neurons.

Isaiah 26:3 "Thou wilt keep him in perfect peace, whose mind is stayed on thee: because he trusteth in thee."

If Heather could sit down and talk with you, she would tell you where her source of strength has come from. She believes that God's Grace is sufficient to all those that put their trust in Him!

If you have not trusted Jesus as your Saviour, please read the following and accept Him without delay! He loves you and longs to give you His Grace to help you day by day!

HERE IS HOW YOU CAN KNOW JESUS AND THE GRACE THAT HE FREELY GIVES

1. EVERYONE IS A SINNER...
"For all have sinned, and come short of the glory of God;" (Romans 3:23) No one is good enough to go to Heaven on his own merit. No matter how much good we do, we still fall short because we were all born into sin.

2. REALIZE THERE IS A PENALTY FOR SIN...
"For the wages of sin is death;..." (Romans 6:23) Just as there are wages for good, there is punishment for wrong. The penalty for our sin is eternal death in a place called Hell.

3. BELIEVE JESUS DIED FOR YOU...
"But God commendeth His love toward us, in that, while we were yet sinners, Christ died for us." (Romans 5:8) Jesus great love was shown for us when He came to the earth and died on the cross to pay for our sin debt. He arose three days later and is alive even now.

HOW YOU CAN KNOW JESUS
(Continued)

4. TRUST CHRIST ALONE AS YOUR SAVIOUR...

"*...But the gift of God is eternal life through Jesus Christ our Lord.*" (Romans 6:23) "*For whosoever shall call upon the name of the Lord shall be saved.*" (Romans 10:13) Everlasting life is a gift purchased by the blood of Jesus and offered freely to those who call upon Him by faith. Trust Jesus by faith to be your Saviour today!

Let us help you word a prayer...
(It's not mere words that save you, but your faith in Jesus Christ.)

"Dear Jesus, I know that I am a sinner. Please forgive me for my sinfulness. Jesus, because you died on the cross for me and rose again, I am now asking you to save my soul from Hell. I place my trust in you, and you alone, to take me to Heaven when I die. Thank you for saving me, Jesus. Amen."

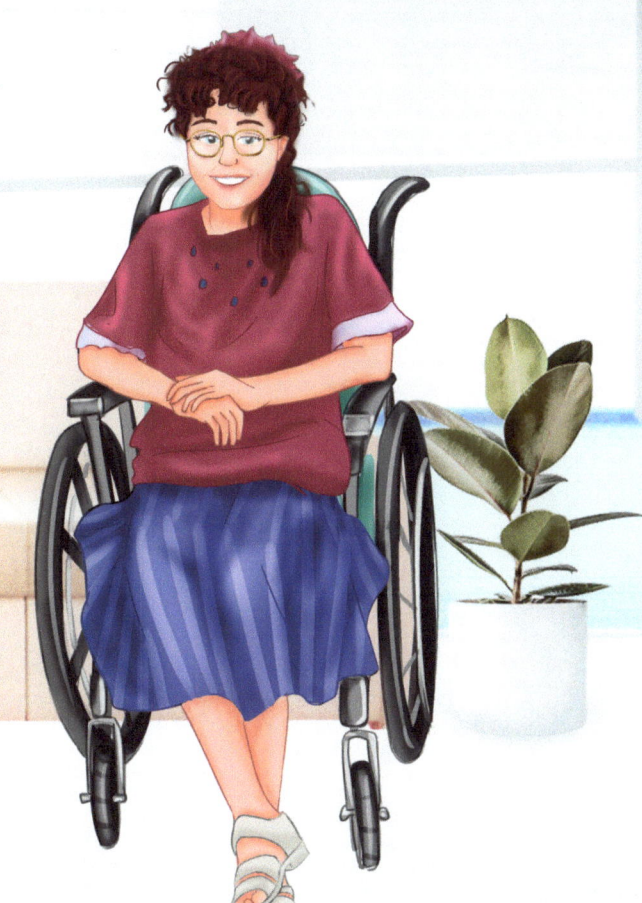

If you just prayed that prayer and accepted Christ into your heart and life, we would love to hear from you. Please contact us at cerebrumconnections@gmail.com.

CEREBRUM CONNECTIONS

Cerebrum Connections is a ministry started to help families engage through medicine and ministry. With 30 years of experience, we are able to help others prepare to work with their doctors, as well as help to direct them to the source of all wisdom and strength, our Lord and Saviour, Jesus Christ.

These resources have been published and more can be found at Godmakesnomistakes.com

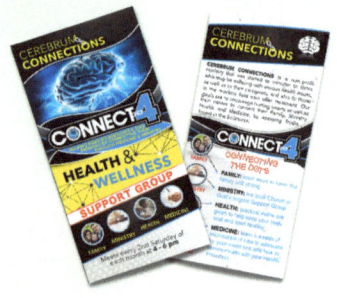
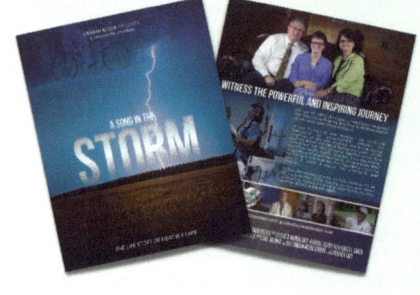
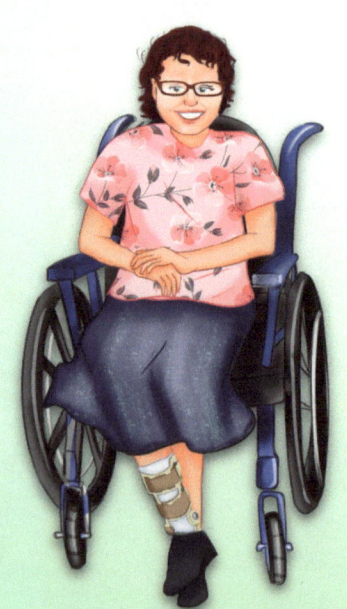
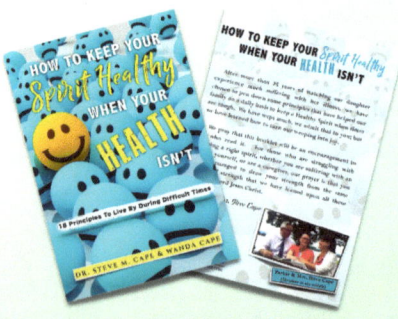
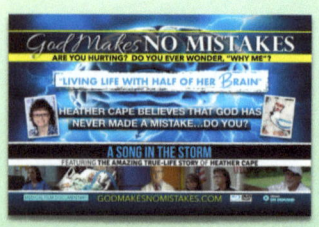

Heather Cape
July 15, 2024

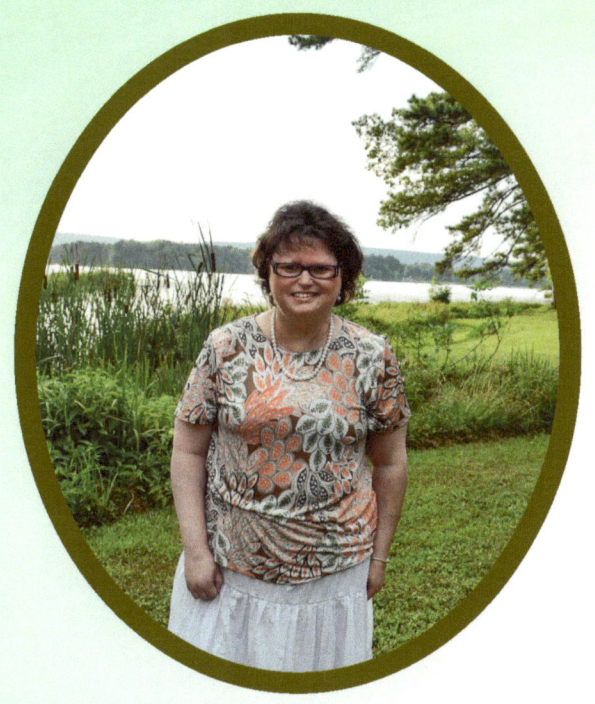

Psalm 59:16-17, "But I will sing of thy power; yea, I will sing aloud of thy mercy in the morning: for thou hast been my defence and refuge in the day of my trouble. Unto thee, O my strength, will I sing: for God is my defence, and the God of my mercy."

It has now been 30 years since that first seizure where Heather's life changed forever. God has used her suffering to speak to the hearts of many people in ways we can't even imagine. It's interesting that she has only one half-of her brain, but, yet, she has accepted her affliction with tremendous grace that can only come from our Heavenly Father. She is very brave and is not afraid to let His light shine through her with everyone she meets. Her strength comes by living from the principles found in the Word of God, as she applies those principles and lives her Christian life every day.

Heather is full of joy and if she ever had trouble thinking of a word, she would often make this statement, "If I only had a brain" and she would chuckle. We decided to change that up a little bit and create this book, "This I Know With Half - Of My Brain".

We have met and continue to meet a lot of hurting people while on this journey. But our Saviour wants to help us all! Most everyone has times when the hardships we face seem to weigh heavy on our hurting hearts, however, our Saviour is waiting to comfort and help us through these troublesome times. Let's give our burdens to Him, and go out and help someone else who is hurting.

www.ingramcontent.com/pod-product-compliance
Lightning Source LLC
Chambersburg PA
CBHW042133070426
42453CB00002BA/77